ALKALINE WATER
WHY YOU NEED IT AND HOW TO GET IT

PATRICIA A. PHILLIPS-WYATT

ISBN: 978-1772770209

PUBLISHED BY:
10-10-10 PUBLISHING
MARKHAM, ON
CANADA

Disclaimer

Contents

Acknowledgements

Most significant achievements in life are the result of collaboration and working with others whose talents and insights enable us to create something new and worthwhile.

To my wonderful husband, David Wyatt, and my children, Boyd Simpson III and Patrice Nicole Brown-Harris, a great big thank you for the support and encouragement throughout this process.

I would like to acknowledge the help and support of my good friend and fellow homeopathic/nutritional advocate, Dr. Gary Strahle, Ph.D, Downey, California. Your encouragement and friendship has been invaluable.

I would also like to acknowledge my two best friends in the healthy water movement, Mr. Michael Maxwell (The Water Man) and his fiancée, Colleen Roberts. With the help of Colleen, my husband and I now have crystal clear well water. Thanks just doesn't seem to be a strong enough word for all the help you have provided us. Love you both dearly.

Raymond Aaron deserves my undying gratitude for coaching me, pushing me and guiding me to finally share my information with the world through writing my books.

Thank you to everyone that reads my book, for giving me the opportunity to share valuable healthy water information with you. Without you this book would not be possible. I have had many questions on what is the best ionizer machine to purchase and why it's even necessary. This book will finally answer your questions so that you can be properly informed.

It is my desire that you discover within these pages the fundamentals of our water sources, to the point that you will put into practice and choose to take into your own hands the quality of the water you drink. This book will change your life forever. Implement what you read and your body will thank you forever.

This book is dedicated to my mother, Mildred L. White-Kaufman (1930-2012) author of "Candid Thoughts In Poetry," Vantage Press 1992.

Mom, your poem "I Can, I Must, I Will" has motivated me and so many of your students to achieve beyond our wildest dreams.

I Can, I Must, I Will

I Can conquer anything that I want
Because
I am bright, I am unique,
And I control my destiny.

I Must,
Because
I own a special place in this universe
And I will not allow anyone
To define my limits
And enclose my boundaries

I Will succeed
Because
I can overcome any obstacle
By using my mind, body, and intellect
To crawl under, walk around,
Or climb over those things
Which hinder me
Because
I Can, I Must, I Will be Successful—
For Me!

Thank you, Mommy

Foreword

Wow, I love the book *"Alkaline Water."* I never knew that pure healthy water was available on this planet anymore.

Whenever I can and whenever it's available to me, that's all that I drink.

I've come to realize the importance of maintaining the proper pH balance in my body. *The Book on Alkaline Water* will educate and inform the reader on this very important issue.

You will learn that most bottled water is actually, in many cases, worse and more expensive than plain tap water.

When I learned that CANCER and disease couldn't survive in an alkaline environment, it became imperative that I keep my body in an alkaline state. Drinking alkaline water is one big step toward that goal.

Patricia's enthusiasm and commitment to researching and sharing this valuable information is commendable and very much appreciated by me. The information in this book has helped me and many others understand the importance of alkaline water in maintaining a healthy internally balanced system for excellent health.

When you really think about it, if you don't have your health, you have nothing.

Raymond Aaron
NY Times Bestselling Author
www.aaron.com

Chapter 1
The History of Our Water

We all know that in the beginning of the earth the waters were clean and pure; there was no pollution or toxins that man had to worry about. That was what was in the beginning; everything was pure, everything was wholesome, and unfortunately this is not the case anymore.

Where we went wrong

Over two thirds of Earth's surface is covered by water; less than a third is taken up by land. As Earth's population continues to grow, people are putting ever-increasing pressure on the planet's water resources. In a sense, our oceans, rivers, and other inland waters are being "squeezed" by human activities—not so they take up less room, but so their quality is reduced. Poorer water quality means water pollution.

We know that pollution is a human problem because it is a relatively recent development in the planet's history: before the 19th century Industrial Revolution, people lived more in harmony with their immediate environment. As industrialization has spread around the globe, so the problem of pollution has spread with it. When Earth's population was much smaller, no one believed pollution would ever present a serious problem. It was once popularly believed that the oceans were far too big to pollute. Today, with around 7 billion people on the planet, it has become apparent that there are limits. Pollution is one of the signs that humans have exceeded those limits.

How serious is the problem? According to the environmental campaign organization World Wildlife Fund (WWF): "Pollution from toxic chemicals threatens life on this planet. Every ocean and every continent, from the tropics to the once-pristine polar regions, is contaminated."

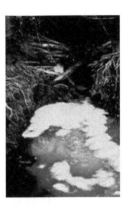

Photo: Detergent pollution entering a river. Photo courtesy of US Fish & Wildlife Service Photo Library.

The Consequence

The consequences of those decisions have been life-threatening. In Arkansas not long ago there were birds falling from the sky, in California recently fish were washing ashore dead. Illness, disease, cancers; all of these things form the consequences of our actions as humans on this earth.

Pollution

Pollutions in our waters, in our streams, have killed animals, killed people and ecosystems. There have been documentaries showing people turning on their water faucets and having their water erupt into flames.

Water pollution almost always means that some damage has been done to an ocean, river, lake, or other water source. A 1969 United Nations report defined ocean pollution as:

"The introduction by man, directly or indirectly, of substances or energy into the marine environment (including estuaries) resulting in such deleterious (harmful) effects as harm to living resources, hazards to human health, hindrance to marine activities, including fishing, impairment of quality for use of sea water and reduction of amenities." [1]

A great deal of water is held in underground rock structures known as aquifers, which we cannot see and seldom think about. Water stored underground in aquifers is known as groundwater. Aquifers feed our rivers and supply much of our drinking water. They too can become polluted, for example, when weed killers used in people's gardens drain into the ground. Groundwater pollution is much less obvious than surface-water pollution, but is no less of a problem. In 1996, a study in Iowa in the United States found that over half the state's groundwater wells were contaminated with weed killers. [2]

Surface waters and groundwater are the two types of water resources that pollution affects. There are also two different ways in which pollution can occur. If pollution comes from a single location, such as a discharge pipe attached to a factory, it is known as point-source pollution. Other examples of point-source pollution include an oil spill from a tanker, a discharge from a smoke stack (factory chimney), or someone pouring oil from their car down a drain. A great deal of water pollution happens not from one single source but from many different scattered sources. This is called nonpoint-source pollution.

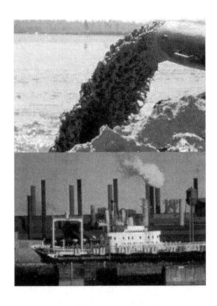

Photo: Above: Point-source pollution comes from a single, well-defined place such as this pipe. Below: Nonpoint-source pollution comes from many sources. All the industrial plants alongside a river and the ships that service them may be polluting the river collectively. Both photos courtesy of US Fish & Wildlife Service Photo Library.

When point-source pollution enters the environment, the place most affected is usually the area immediately around the source. For example, when a tanker accident occurs, the oil slick is concentrated around the tanker itself and, in the right ocean conditions, the pollution disperses the further away from the tanker you go. This is less likely to happen with nonpoint-source pollution which, by definition, enters the environment from many different places at once.

Sometimes pollution that enters the environment in one place has an effect hundreds or even thousands of miles away. This is known as trans-boundary pollution. One example is the way radioactive waste travels through the oceans from nuclear reprocessing plants in England and France to nearby countries such as Ireland and Norway.

- Residue of food additives and agrochemicals significantly contaminates our bodily fluids.
- 80% of newborns have allergies, caused by mothers' tainted body fluids.

Sources & References:
Water: http://www.explainthatstuff.com/water.html
Rivers: http://www.www.explainthatstuff.com/rivers.html
1. http://www.Explainthatstuff.com/waterpollution.html #gesampfn
2. http://www. Explainthatstuff.com/waterpollution.html

Chapter 2
What is Alkaline/Ionized Mineral Water?

We hear a lot about the problems citizens of this country are faced with when it comes to polluted water these days. Many are left with few options when it comes to avoiding drinking polluted or contaminated water.

The recent disaster in Flint, Michigan is cause for all of us to take notice and give some serious thought to this most important element to our lives (water). It was discovered recently that exorbitant amounts of lead, (see: http://cnn.it/1SJn6XG and http://www.huffingtonpost.com/ entry/flint-michigan-water-lead_us_56784055e460b958f657595c) are in the municipal water supplies and not that long ago water pollution problems where discovered in West Virginia (Jan. 2014) (See: http://www.nytimes.com/2014/01/11/us/west-virginia-chemical-spill.html?_r=1) . Even in my home state of North Carolina pollution of our rivers and streams with Coal Ash are polluting the water table putting all of us at risk. See www.southeastcoalash.org

Who is responsible for the quality of the water we drink? Who is going to pay the medical bills of the injured children and residents of these communities who have been stricken with lead exposure as a result of drinking this tainted water?

In this chapter I'm going to provide you with a definition of what Alkaline/Ionized water is as well as information on how the purification of your water can be achieved. This method takes a little effort on your part but still is a viable addition or alternative to an actual Ionizer machine. This mineral additive is called, **black mica.**

I know it will seem odd that with all the information I'm going to provide about Alkaline/Ionizer machines, that I would spend so much time discussing a purification process that has existed since the beginning of time. But; with all the pollution being experienced by so many citizens, purification processes that go above and beyond are warranted.

Alkaline/Ionizer machines aide in the process of restoring your body to an alkaline state. If your body is acidic you are at risk of several maladies that will be discussed in later chapters.

Black Mica, however, like some high-end Ionizer machines, can remove contaminants such as:

1. Hazardous heavy metals, Mercury, Lead, Arsenic, and harmful Aluminum.
2. Toxic chemicals: Sodium Fluoride, Chlorine and its byproducts, 80 volatile organic compounds, and Chromium-6.
3. BPAs, PCBs, Phthalates and other substances that damage your hormone system.
4. Pathogenic bacteria and viruses.
5. Agricultural chemicals: pesticides, herbicide, and fungicides.

It appears that the book "Alkaline Water, Why You Need It and How To Get It", is very timely indeed.

Clean Water

Clean mineralized water is needed for the sustainability of all life on earth. Clean water full of all the natural mineral nutrients that come with it are what we need as humans. Mineral rich water provides the nutrients that we all need.

Alkaline/Ionized Water

Water at its purest level is comprised of molecules that have two hydrogen atoms and one oxygen atom. Because there are generally minerals in drinking water, a hydrogen atom can split off from the molecule. When it does, it has a positive charge and is called an ion. The remaining hydrogen and oxygen atoms have a net negative charge. Because positive and negative charges are attracted to each other, any hydrogen atom that breaks off will generally combine with another hydrogen-oxygen pair to form a water molecule again. Alkaline/Ionized water has a higher concentration of hydrogen atoms, or ions, than normal drinking water.

Alkaline/Ionized water takes us back to where we were in the beginning, and the Alkaline/Ionized water machine does exactly that. It gives you the internal balance that you need. The right pH balance within your body is what will help to ward off many diseases. That is the Alkaline/Ionized water difference.

Alkaline/Ionized water is delicious water created from innovative water technology. Not only do these devices filter your tap water, but they also produce Alkaline/Ionized alkaline and acidic waters through electrolysis. These waters can be used for various purposes, including drinking, cooking, beauty, and cleaning.

The Facts

- Alkaline/Ionized water can have higher concentrations of hydrogen atoms, or positive ions, in which case it would be called acidic. Alkaline/Ionized water with higher concentrations of the hydrogen-oxygen pairs is called alkaline. There are consumer machines that ionize water and some that will separate water into these two types of Alkaline/Ionized water and/or Alkaline and Acidic water. I use the acidic component to disinfect and clean my home.

- There is another modality that can be employed to achieve the elimination of heavy metals, chemicals and microorganisms. This is known scientifically as Biotite. *Biotite or **black mica**, K(Mg,Fe2+)3(Al,Fe3+)Si3O10(OH,F)2, is rich in iron and magnesium and typically occurs in mafic igneous rocks).*

  o Biotite is so common that it's considered a rock-forming mineral. Biotite is named in honor of Jean Baptiste Biot, a French physicist who first described the optical effects in the mica minerals. Biotite actually is a range of black micas; depending on their iron content they range from eastonite through siderophyllite to phlogopite. If you aren't a mineral fanatic, ignore all that.

  o Biotite occurs widely throughout many different rock types, adding glitter to schist, "pepper" in salt-and-pepper granite, and darkness to sandstones. This is a powerful combination of the earth's naturally occurring minerals including iron, potassium and magnesium. Through a proprietary process (U.S. patent 4,776,963), black mica is extracted for water purification. In the U.S., Adya Clarity™ is registered and marketed for water purification.

This is what we really want and need. Alkaline/Ionized mineral water!

Let's take a look at some of these very dangerous contaminants eliminated by using either a high end ionizer and/or Adya Clarity™.

Serious Dangers Caused by the Contaminants

1. Heavy Metals

Lead- One of the Most Lethal Metals

Lead pollutes water through corrosion of old pipes, the built-in water service lines for water delivery from the source to the homes. This is very common if you live in an older city.

The Environmental Working Group warns the public about the dangers of Lead, even "low doses matter".

The American Journal of Cardiology and the American Medical Association both confirm that heavy metal toxicity is directly correlated with cardiovascular diseases and cancer.

Trace amounts of lead are also found to cause negative changes in human behavior. Specifically, lead exposure in children causes severe damage to their physical and mental development, resulting in learning disabilities, hearing loss, delinquency, attention deficits, mental disturbances, and lowered IQ. This damage is permanent and irreversible.

Lead in drinking water may also contribute to many other adverse health effects in adults such as increased blood pressure, chronic kidney disease, and negative neurobehavioral changes.

Mercury- Extremely Potent, Invisible & Odorless, Neurotoxin

Mercury is a powerful neurotoxin that affects all of your vital organs and the entire nervous system. Over exposure to Mercury can result in muscle twitches and digestive issues, leading to more severe conditions like neurological issues, autoimmune diseases, severe allergic reactions and even mental disorders such as dementia and Parkinson's. It can even build up in your spinal fluid and travel into a fetus via the placenta.

Aluminum- Brain Degenerative Poison

The Global Healing Center reports that chronic Aluminum exposure can cause skeletal deformities, brain degeneration, and nervous system disorders Aluminum begins to accumulate in your body, builds up in vital organs and tissues, and disrupts your body's normal biological functioning. Symptoms of Aluminum toxicity can range anywhere from minor physical ailments such as headaches or forgetfulness to chronic conditions such a liver and kidney damage and Alzheimer's disease.

Arsenic- Deadly Runoff Contaminant

The major source of Arsenic in drinking water is due to runoff from agricultural and industrial practices and from the erosion of natural Arsenic-rich rock deposits. Studies done by both the US Environmental Protection Agency (EPA) and the National Academy of Sciences report that Arsenic in drinking water may cause cancer in the bladder, lung, skin, kidney, liver, prostate, and nasal passages. Arsenic may also damage the central and peripheral nervous systems, the heart and blood vessels, as well as serious skin problems and birth defects. The EPA also warns the public of Arsenic's non-cancer negative effects which includes the thickening and discoloration of the skin, stomach pain, nausea, vomiting, diarrhea, numbness in hands and feet, partial paralysis, and even blindness.

2. Chemicals

Fluoride- Industrial Bi-Product & Deadly Neurotoxin

Fluoride is one of the most difficult water contaminants to remove. Among damaging your bones, joints, and brain, fluoride may also destruct your immune system, thyroid function, DNA, and has even been shown to cause cancerous tumors. A study published by Harvard University funded by the National Institute of Health Research has concluded that children who live in areas with highly fluoridated water have "significantly lower" IQ scores than those who live in low fluoride areas. To make matters worse, fluoridated water increases the body's absorption of heavy metals.

Chlorine and its byproducts - Carcinogenic War Weapon

To remove pathogens and microorganisms, water treatment plants add chlorine, chloramine and other chemical disinfectant to "sanitize" our water. However, the residual chlorine often leaves a "chemical" smell to our water. Chlorine also reacts with organic matter creating deadly compounds called Trihalomethanes (THMs) and Haloacetic acids (HAA5s). These disinfectant byproducts are 100 times more toxic than chlorine itself and have long been known as carcinogenic and neurotoxic. The U.S. Council of Environmental Quality admits that drinking chlorinated water increases your cancer risk by a whopping 93%. Recognizing the danger of chlorine, water treatment plants have switched from chlorine to chloramines. However, recent evidence suggests that chloramines may increase the amount of dissolved lead in water.

Chromium-6- The "Erin Brokovich" Contaminant

Hexavalent Chromium is a toxic metal produced by industrial processes and manufacturing activities such as discharges from steel and pulp mills. Chromium-6 is carcinogenic in drinking water and at least 74 million Americans in 42 states are drinking Chromium-6 polluted tap water.

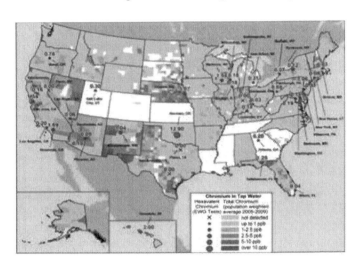

3. Microorganisms

Human and animal wastes foster the growth of microorganisms. When present in high volumes, the chemical disinfectants added to our water are not sufficient to kill them. In addition, many of these pathogens have become highly resistant to current disinfection practices. Heat can be one way used to kill pathogens that cause water borne diseases. However boiling your water increases the concentration of nitrates and heavy metals that may cause serious health effects.

Findings:

- According to 2008 study published by the New York Times, about 19.5 million people in the United States get sick from microorganisms in water every year.

- A study released by the American Journal of Public Health estimates that 35% of gastrointestinal diseases are caused by drinking contaminated tap water.

- World Health Organization reported that approximately 1.8 million people die annually from pathogenic microorganisms and waterborne diseases.

- From 2009 –2010, untreated ground water deficiencies and distribution systems deficiencies such as leaky pipes are responsible for 24% and 12% of outbreak-associated illnesses, respectively.

- There are 300,000 water main breaks in the United States each year, which means there is one water main break every 2 minutes. The problem is that our entire water infrastructure is crumbling.

Adya Clarity™ removes these odorless and tasteless toxins lurking in your water.

What is Adya Clarity™?

Adya Clarity™ is a blend of purified water and ionic sulfate minerals extracted from **black mica** that provides a simple yet revolutionary way to detoxify your water. Without the use of toxic, synthetic chemicals, it removes harmful contaminants and delivers a pure, refreshing taste to your water.

Even though I personally enjoy the ease of allowing my ionizer machine to do all the work for me I would be remise if I didn't introduce an addition to or alternative to the ionizer machine. I found it in Adya Clarity™.

Adya Clarity™ as a Water Purification Tool

The ionic sulfate minerals in Adya Clarity™ activate water's natural ability to filter out chemical and biological contaminants. After this purification process, water is turned back to its clean, pristine, and primordial state; hence, the name of the product: Adya (Ah-Dee-YA), which means "primordial", or the "original, best state" in Sanskrit (classical language of Indian).

The Science Behind Adya Clarity™

1. Water purification

Adya Clarity™ contains ionic sulphate minerals that have anionic and cationic exchange properties - the ability to donate or receive electrons. It activates water's natural ability to cleanse itself from chemical and biological contaminants.

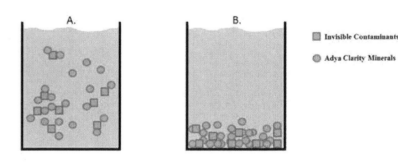

2. Forming Stable and Balanced Minerals

Adya Clarity™ contains ionic sulfate minerals, which are powerful ions that can break up the bonds of weak but harmful minerals. Because a balance of minerals is present in Adya Clarity™, ions are rearranged to form strong and stable mineral bonds. For example, when Adya Clarity™ is added to water, Sodium Fluoride, a toxic mineral salt which has a relatively weak bond, converts to Calcium Fluoride, a harmless mineral salt that appears naturally in underground water sources and in seawater.

3. Keeping Your Water Fresh and Clean

Adya Clarity™ activates oxygen that breaks down waste and neutralizes contaminants so that they are no longer toxic. The activated oxygen also kills disease-causing microorganisms, and prevents bacterial growth. So the harmful contaminants that make your water rot cannot grow in water.

4. Lab Results – Benefits Proven by Science

Adya Clarity™ has been:

- Tested and proven by the Environmental Protection Agency (EPA) certified lab results. Results are available at http://www.adyawater.com/pages/adya-clarity-lab-tests
- Tested and proven by 2 separate human clinical trials. Available here: http://www.waterliberty.com/pdfs/Heavy_Metal_30-day_study.pdf http://waterliberty.com/pdfs/Heavy-Metal-90-Day-Final-21.pdf

Brief Summary of Water Purification Benefits

Adya Clarity™:

- Reduces 159 harmful industrial chemicals including 80 volatile organic compounds.
- Removes 100% of chlorine and reduces chloramines and trihalomethanes to undetectable limits.
- Reduces 99.95% of tested pharmaceuticals and basic drugs.
- Reduces 79 different agricultural substances.
- Reduces heavy metals in water including Lead, Arsenic, and Mercury to undetectable limits.
- Converts toxic Chromium-6 in water to beneficial Chromium-3, an essential dietary element.
- Converts toxic Sodium Fluoride in water to harmless Calcium Fluoride, which naturally occurs in various water sources.
- Kills 4 types of disease causing microorganisms and prevents their growth.
- Reduces up to 99.85% of tested bacteria, viruses, and parasites.
- Provides up to 100 trace minerals that are easily absorbed by the body.

On a molecular level all the trillions of cells in your body are actually composed of 99.9% water. Looking inside the cells, you are basically 99.9% water. You're not a body containing water; you are water in the form of a human being.

The water you're drinking really deserves a second look.

Did you know that water could actually store energetic information? Water is the most mysterious substance on the planet. It is the key to life and it does things that even defy the laws of physics. Think about this...have you ever wondered how water defies the laws of gravity to send nourishment to the top of the tallest trees and its branches?

Water has structure, most of us know the structures of solid (ice), gas (steam), and liquid which has a huge impact on how your cells interact with nutrients and proteins. But, there is a 4th structure.

The cells in your body are surrounded by mostly water, and there is now a mountain of evidence, which proves the type of water you drink is possibly the most important element of health **because it changes how your cells absorb nutrients, and how they behave (the 4th structure).**

Let's stop for a moment and think about what happens to a gold fish that's been swimming around in unchanged water for a couple of weeks. Many of us have seen this scenario. You come home one day and your poor gold fish is upside down in the tank. Was the gold fish sick or the water? If the water had been changed on a regular basis more than likely the gold fish would have survived. It's the same for us as humans. If you change the environment in your body you can change the physiological state of your body.

To be honest we are pretty screwed in terms of our water supply and our environment. See chapter 5 to see some of what is allowed, by FDA and the Safe Water Drinking Act mandate, in our water supply right now.

So what can be done to get our bodies back to a normal pH balance? There is something we can do. As I've written about, previously in this book, using Adya Clarity™ and/or a quality ionizer will infuse your tap or well water with the necessary oxygen and minerals to accomplish the task of achieving Alkaline/Ionized Mineral water.

If you don't mind waiting a few hours you can add "**Black Mica** extract" (Adya Clarity™) to your tap water and achieve Mineral water. With the "Black Mica extract" the unwanted chemicals, heavy metals, pharmaceuticals and bacteria are bound and clumped together at the bottom of your container making them non-effective and inert. You can use a coffee filter to remove them if you like.

Remember, just because you can't see the contaminants doesn't mean they're not there.

The minerals found in "**Black Mica**" (Adya Clarity™) are usually found near slow moving volcanic eruptions...they come from deep within the earth. This is why you normally only find them in the water that comes from natural hot springs and mineral springs, which are found near volcanoes.

Healing Hot Springs and Mineral Springs

- Hot Springs and Mineral Springs are known to extract toxins out of the body.
- Used for thousands of years to reverse disease in ways modern science is just beginning to understand.

This is the key to healing water and restoring its healing properties.

Adya Clarity™ as a Natural Health Product

1. Effective in Prevention and Opportunity to Heal

Adya Clarity™ is filled with ionic sulphate minerals that protect you from the harmful contaminants in your water. Adya Clarity™ makes these contaminants inert. Without the constant exposure to these poisons your body will have time to recoup and heal. As a result, common chronic health conditions and symptoms of toxicity will often ease up or completely disappear after the regular intake of the purified Adya Clarity™ water.

2. Remove Toxin Buildup From Your Body

Adya Clarity™ has been clinically proven to be safe for human consumption. It is also proven that the same purifying effect is noticeable inside our body since a human body is composed of 70-99.9% water. Adya Clarity™ has been found to be effective in heavy metal removal from the body by an average of 82% in 90 days. These toxic metals include Aluminum, Mercury, Lead, and Arsenic. Additionally, hydration of the cells was improved by 32%. See the human trial studies at. http://waterliberty.com/pdfs/Heavy-Metal-90-Day-Final-21.pdf

Instructions For Use

Conversions:

1. How Much Adya Clarity™ Should Be Used

The amount depends on the quality and type of water. Generally, the more contaminants that are in the water, the more Adya Clarity™ is needed to purify your water.

For most water it is recommended that you start with a dilution ration of 1:1000

To calculate the amount of Adya Clarity™ you need to divide the volume of water by 1000.

Example: (1 liter of water/1000= 1ml of Adya Clarity=1/5
teaspoon = 20 drops
1 teaspoon = 100 drops

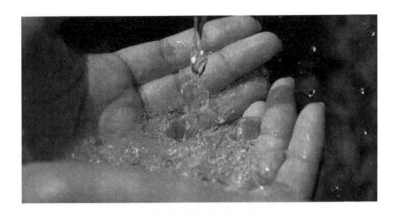

2. To Purify Large Amounts of Drinking Water

Recommended dosage per 1.3 gallon (5 liters) of water.

Type of Water	Recommended Dosage per 1.3 gallons (5 liters) of Water
Tap Water	
Well Water	1-2 teaspoons
Filtered Water	
Spring Water	1 teaspoon
Distilled Water	
Reverse Osmosis Water	1/2 teaspoon

3. To Purify Smaller Amounts of Drinking Water

For most water, it is recommended to add 5-8 drops for every 8 oz. of water.

- For distilled or Reverse Osmosis water (which is generally clean but is lacking the minerals), reduce the dosage by half, from5-8 drops to 2-4 drops for every 8 oz. This enhances the water with essential minerals.

Volume of Water	Recommended Dosage
8oz (237ml)	5-8 drops
16oz (473ml)	10-16 drops
32oz (946ml) (1 quart)	20-32 drops

Treatment Process

1. What Should Be Done After Adding Adya Clarity™ To My Drinking Water?

- Stir to ensure contaminants are binding to the minerals in Adya Clarity™
- Keep the lid off or cover loosely to allow gaseous contaminants such as Chlorine and other chemicals, volatile by-products to evaporate.
- Wait while treating water at room temperature. Do not refrigerate water during treatment because cold temperatures slow precipitation.

2. How Long Do I Wait Before Drinking The Water?

The wait time depends on the quality of the original water. Longer wait time ensures all complex contaminants, such as micro-organisms, are removed.

If you are confident that the starting water is clean (i.e. distilled and reverse osmosis water), wait 5-15 minutes before drinking. For polluted water, the suggested wait time is 24-72 hours.

*Time Saving Tips:

1. Treat two large batches of water at a time. When one batch of water is still being treated, you can drink the batch that is already purified.
2. Adding Adya Clarity™ to warm or hot water would speed up the purification process.

Sources & References

Rock Forming Mineral:
http://geology.about.com/od/minerals/ig/minpicrockforming/

Phlogopite:
http://geology.about.com/od/minerals/ig/minpicmicas/minipic
phlogopite.htm

Schist:
http://geology.about.com/od/rocks/ig/metrockindex/rocpicshis
t.htm

Granite:
http://geology.about.com/od/rocks/ig/igrockindex/rocpicgranit
e.htm

Chapter 3
What Is An Alkalizing Diet?

An alkalizing diet is a diet that emphasizes, to a varying degree, fresh fruit, vegetables, roots and tubers, nuts, and legumes. It is also known as the "alkalizing acid diet".

History

In alternative medicine, the alkalizing diet is based on the belief that our hunter-gatherer ancestors consumed a diet very different than what is consumed today. The diet was based on minimally processed plant and animal foods.

With the advent of modern agriculture, the standard Western diet changed greatly.

- Grains were introduced into the diet after the appearance of stone tools. Refined grains were available after the invention of automated rolling and sifting devices.
- Milk, cheese and other milk products were introduced with the domestication of livestock.
- Salt consumption rose when technology to mine, process, and transport it became available.
- Meat consumption increased with animal husbandry. It further increased with the advent of technology that enabled grains to be efficiently fed to cattle, which allowed cattle to be fattened quickly.
- Sugar consumption has risen since the beginning of the Industrial Revolution.

According to alkalizing diet proponents, almost all foods that we eat release either an acid or an alkalizing base (bicarbonate) into blood after being digested, absorbed, and metabolized. Grains, fish, meat, poultry, shellfish, cheese, milk, and salt all produce acid, so the introduction and dramatic rise in our consumption of these foods meant that the typical Western diet became more acid-producing.

Our blood is slightly alkaline, with normal pH level of between 7.35 and 7.45. The belief behind the alkalizing diet is that our diet should reflect this pH level (as it did in the past) and be slightly alkaline.

Proponents of alkalizing diets believe that a diet high in acid-producing foods disrupts this balance and promotes the loss of essential minerals such as potassium, magnesium, calcium, and sodium, as the body tries to restore equilibrium. This imbalance is thought to make people prone to illness.

Why Do People Try the Alkalizing Diet?

According to some alternative practitioners, the shift to an acid-producing diet is linked to a number of chronic illnesses and symptoms.

- Lack of energy
- Excessive mucous production
- Nasal congestion
- Frequent colds and flu
- Anxiety, nervousness, irritability
- Ovarian cysts, polycystic ovaries, benign breast cysts
- Headaches

Although conventional medical doctors generally agree that a plant-based diet with an abundance of fruit and vegetables and minimal salt and refined grains is beneficial to health, conventional doctors do not believe that an acid-producing diet is the foundation of chronic illness. In conventional medicine, there is evidence, however, that some of the foods allowed on the alkalizing diet may improve overall health.

Caveats

The alkalizing diet should not be used by people with kidney failure or cancer unless under a doctor's supervision. People with heart disease and those on medications that affect potassium levels in the body should check with their doctor first.

The alkalizing diet hasn't been tested for safety; and keep in mind that the safety of the diet in pregnant women, nursing mothers, children, and those with medical conditions or who are taking medications has not been established. If you're considering trying an alkalizing diet, talk with your primary care provider first.

Sources:

Cordain L, Eaton SB, Sebastian A, Mann N, Lindeberg S, Watkins BA, O'Keefe JH, Brand-Miller J. Origins and Evolution of the Western Diet: health implications for the 21st Century. American Journal of Clinical Nutrition. 81.2 (2005): 341-354.

Minich DM, Bland JS. Acid-alkalizing balance: role in chronic disease and detoxification.

Alternative Therapies in Health and Medicine. 13.4 (2007): 62-65

Read More: http://www.ehow.com/about_5033313_alkalizing-water.html

Chapter 4
The Bottled Water Misconception

Why is Bottled Water Better; Or is it?

Here are some important facts that I feel you should consider and be aware of:

- Municipal filtration systems do not provide us pure water with the necessary minerals that our bodies need on a consistent basis.
- Believe it or not, most bottled water is very acidic, which in turn causes rapid oxidation within our bodies (thus the need to consume antioxidants to counter this phenomenon). I have personally tested most of the brands on the market today and they most all test out in the high acidic range. See www.kangendemo.com
- Some bottled water claims to use a system of Reverse Osmosis. This a system by which everything is removed from the water. Every nutritional component is stripped from the water. You are left with nothing but dead water with no beneficial properties to it at all.
- Water softener systems are good if you have very hard water coming into your home. Be aware that these systems add salts and other chemicals to achieve the goal of softer water.
- Landfills are filled with the plastic from bottled water along with other trash that doesn't break down. When exposed to the elements, poisons are released and end up in our water supplies.
- Plastics do not break down on our planet, and not only that but most plastic water bottles are produced using petroleum by-products.

The Petroleum Influence

Petroleum by-products are used to create the bottles that bottled water is placed in.

Polyethylene Terephthalate

Polyethylene terephthalate (PET), being a lightweight but strong plastic, is broadly used in the packaging industry, such as in plastic bottles. According to Food and Drug Administration (FDA), "PET makes up 6.5 percent of all carbonated beverage and water bottles." It is resistant to the effects of damage of chemicals and moisture, also possessing good insulating properties. PET is also used in products such as cable wraps, transformer insulation, generator parts, and polyester fabrics.

Natural Gas and Oil

Natural gas and oil are considered the primary raw materials in plastic production. The first procedure in plastic production is the "cracking" of natural gas or crude oil. The "cracking process" refers to the conversion of crude oil or natural gas into hydrocarbon monomers. These monomers include propylene and ethylene. In some cases, the cracking process converts crude oil or natural gas into other monomers including: terephthatic acid, styrene, ethylene glycol, vinyl chloride and similar components. Afterward, the hydrocarbon monomers go through a chemical process that helps them bind together. Depending on the kind of plastic to be produced, these monomers may be manipulated to bond in different ways. The resulting product, polymers, may go through further processes to create distinct plastic products with specific functions.

Plasticizers

Plastics have two distinct components: polymers from natural gas or oil, and additives. At present, the most common type of additives used in plastic production is plasticizers. Plasticizers are responsible for the durable and flexible characteristics of plastics. Plasticizers hold a comparatively large market in the plastic additives industry. Other applications of plasticizers include production of: polyvinyl chloride (PVC), plastic bottles, and plumbing products, coating and even in construction materials. While a range of chemicals may be used as plasticizers, phthalates is the most widely used. Because of rising environmental concerns, another alternative to phthalates as plasticizer is now being used, and that is none other than vegetable oil.

What are the effects of heating and or freezing water bottles?

Although I could find no credible information suggesting that doing so would cause the leaching of harmful production ingredients, it only makes sense not to chance it.

Ever noticed the after-taste that seems to exist with most bottled water?

Bottled Water vs. Tap Water

According to the United Nations, 783 million people worldwide – nearly one out of every nine people in the world – don't have reliable access to clean water. One of the worst countries for water access is the tiny island nation of Fiji, where, as reporter Charles Fishman told NPR in 2010, nearly 53% of the population doesn't have a clean, safe source of drinking water.

Ironically, Fiji is also the home of the plant that bottles Fiji Water, one of the most popular brands of bottled water in the United States. Americans, unlike Fijians, have no shortage of safe water to drink – the Safe Drinking Water Act (SDWA) holds all public sources of drinking water to strict safety standards, ensuring that the vast majority of U.S. citizens can trust the water that comes out of their tap. Even so, many Americans choose to pass over this abundant clean water source in favor of bottled waters.

Americans have many reasons to prefer bottled water to tap water. Some just don't care for the taste of their local tap water; others like the convenience of a portable, disposable bottle. Whatever their reasons, they're part of a large and growing trend. Statistics from the International Bottled Water Association (IBWA) show that Americans consumed 10.9 billion gallons of bottled water in 2014 – 34.2 gallons for every man, woman, and child in the country.

But all this bottled water comes with a cost – both for consumers and for the environment. Bottled water is far more expensive than tap water, and it also uses many more resources to package, ship, and dispose of when the bottles are empty. These costs have many people wondering whether it's time to lose the ubiquitous water bottle and go back to tap water.

The Rise of Bottled Water

Bottled water has grown more and more popular over the last few decades. The IBWA estimates that in 1976, each American drank 1.6 gallons of bottled water. By 2014, they were drinking more than 21 times as much. Today, more than one out of every six bottled drinks sold in this country is a bottle of water, making bottled water nearly as popular as carbonated soft drinks.

The IBWA attributes the growing popularity of bottled water to health-consciousness. A 16-ounce bottle of Coca-Cola has 190 calories and 52 grams of sugar, while a 16-ounce bottle of water has no calories, no sugar, and no artificial sweeteners. However, that doesn't explain why consumers are choosing bottled water over tap water, which is also sugar-free and calorie-free.

When reporters ask consumers why they prefer bottled water, they get a variety of answers:

- **Taste**. Many New Yorkers interviewed by ABC News in 2005 said they chose bottled water because it tasted better. One woman described her favorite bottled water as "crisp" and "natural," while another complained that tap water "kind of tastes like sewer." In general, consumers described the local tap water as flat and flavorless.

- **Health**. Other interviewees in the ABC News story believed bottled water was safer or healthier than tap water. One man said he was the only one in his family "brave enough" to drink the local tap water. Everyone else was afraid it would be full of germs. Another man said he felt "more comfortable" giving his young daughter bottled water.

- **Convenience**. Many users find bottled water more convenient than tap water, especially when they're away from home. Instead of having to look for a water fountain when they get thirsty, they can just grab a bottle of water on their way out the door, or pick one up at any convenience store. Some people even keep a case of water bottles in the trunk of the car, where they're always at the ready.

- **Fashion**. To many people, bottled water – especially the hip, upscale brands – is trendy and cool. Perrier, the first bottled water to become popular in the USA, built its reputation on being the beverage of choice for upwardly mobile city dwellers. Today, with dozens of different bottled waters to choose from, the bottle you carry can be a fashion statement, just like your shoes or sunglasses.

Tap Water vs. Bottled

The perceived benefits of bottled water aren't always accurate. In most places, tap water is just as safe to drink as bottled water – and, according to blind taste tests, just as tasty as well. And while bottled water can indeed be more convenient and trendy than tap water, it's also more expensive and wasteful. Here's a look at how tap water and bottled water stack up on four major criteria: cost, taste, safety, and sustainability.

Cost

Bottled water isn't just more expensive than tap water – it's a lot more expensive. According to the IBWA, the average cost per gallon of bottled water – not counting imported or sparkling waters – was $1.21 in 2013. That doesn't sound too bad until you look at the cost of tap water, which is $2 per every thousand gallons, according to the U.S. Environmental Protection Agency (EPA). That means that, priced by the gallon, bottled water is more than 600 times more expensive than tap water.

That's only the average price, however. It factors in all the "bottled" water that's delivered in jugs to office buildings or sold in large, refillable containers. However, according to the Beverage Marketing Corporation, about 65% of all bottled water sales come from single-serve plastic bottles, which cost a lot more per gallon. If you spend $1 on a 16.9-ounce bottle of water, you're effectively paying $7.57 per gallon – 3,785 times more than you'd pay for the same amount of water from a faucet.

Spending $1 on a bottle of water every now and then isn't that big a deal, but when you make a regular habit of it, it really adds up. If you buy just one $1 bottle of water each day, your annual spending on bottled water comes to $365. Getting the same amount of water from your tap would cost you less than $0.10.

Moreover, when you pay a price premium for bottled water, what you're getting is often just tap water that's been filtered or purified in some way. Both Dasani, bottled by the Coca-Cola company, and Aquafina, bottled by PepsiCo, start out with public water sources. If filtered tap water is what you want, for about $40 – less than the cost of six weeks' worth of bottled water – you could install a simple faucet-mounted filter in your kitchen and make your own.

Taste

One of the most common reasons people give for drinking bottled water is that it tastes better than their local tap water. For instance, in a blind taste test at the offices of Buzzfeed, staffers universally agreed that all the bottled waters they tried were better than the sample of unfiltered Los Angeles tap water, which tasters described as "pool water" and "disgusting."

However, this result is actually the exception rather than the norm. In most blind taste tests, tap water easily holds its own against bottled waters, even the pricey ones. You can see the same result in numerous cities, both in the U.S. and abroad:

- New York City. In a 2005 taste test run by the ABC News show 20/20, New York City tap water came in tied for third out of six water samples. Even users who said they didn't like tap water had no problem with it when they didn't know what it was. And in an earlier test, run by ABC's Good

Morning America, tap water actually trounced the competition, beating out three other waters – including the high-end imported brand Evian, which almost no one liked.

- Boston. In 2011, Boston University conducted a blind taste test to compare tap water with Vermont Pure bottled water, the brand used in the student lounge's water cooler. Dozens of students sampled both waters and were asked to guess which was which. Of the 67 testers, only one-third of the respondents correctly identified the tap water sample. Another one-third thought it was the bottled water, and the rest said they couldn't tell the difference.

- Washington, D.C. The Center for Nutrition, Diet and Health at the University of the District of Columbia conducted a blind taste test with 218 participants, most of whom said they preferred to drink bottled water at home. Testers tried samples of four waters – tap water, spring water, distilled water, and mineral water – and ranked them in order of preference. Tap water wasn't the top pick, but it came in a close second, with 30% of the vote.

- Cleveland. ABC's NewsChannel5 Cleveland invited residents to try samples of three waters: Sam's Choice Purified bottled water from Walmart, Aquafina bottled water, and Cleveland tap water. Once again, tap water wasn't the favorite, but it came in a close second to Aquafina. Both samples were preferred by more than two to one over the Sam's Choice water – which most people guessed was tap water.

- San Francisco. In 2009, testers at Mother Jones magazine compared samples of their local San Francisco tap water – both filtered and unfiltered – with samples of eight different bottled waters. The unfiltered tap water came in third, beating out expensive brands such as Voss, Evian, and Fiji Water. Interestingly, the filtered tap water was far lower down the list. Tasters found it "tinny and metallic."

- Belfast, Ireland. In a BBC News story, passersby on a Belfast street were invited to try samples of three different waters. The first, "harvested from icebergs in the Canadian Arctic," sells for more than 26 pounds – about $40 – per bottle; the second, made from the sap of maple trees, costs the equivalent of $24; and the third came from the tap. Most tasters couldn't correctly identify the tap water, and one described the $40 sample as "horrible."

Even in southern California, where the Buzzfeed staff found the tap water so dreadful, many consumers think it tastes great – as long as it's served in a fancy bottle. A popular YouTube video shows an elaborate con run by stage magicians Penn and Teller in a "very trendy California restaurant," where they created a phony "water list" of six different imported bottled waters selling for as much as $7 per bottle.

In reality, all six bottles – from "Mount Fuji" to "L'eau Du Robinet," which is French for "tap water" – were filled with a garden hose on the patio. Restaurant patrons claimed to be able to taste distinct differences among the various brands, and consistently agreed that they were much better than tap water – which is exactly what they all were.

Safety

Many people choose bottled water because of concerns about the safety of their tap water. In many cases, these fears are perfectly reasonable.

Environmental writer Elizabeth Royte, author of the new book, *Bottlemania: How Water Went on Sale and Why We Bought It*, points out in an interview with NPR that more than 10% of the community water systems in the U.S. don't meet the standards set by the Safe Drinking Water Act. Also, about 10% of all Americans get their water from private wells, which aren't covered under the SDWA. That means about 60 million Americans are getting tap water that may or may not be safe to drink.

However, choosing bottled water isn't really a solution. According to the EPA, the standards for bottled water in the U.S. are exactly the same as those for tap water – and bottled water isn't subject to the same reporting standards as tap water. Under the SDWA, municipal water systems must send users a consumer confidence report once per year telling them where their water comes from and whether it meets federal standards.

Bottled water, by contrast, is considered a food product and regulated by the Food and Drug Administration (FDA). Under FDA rules, bottled water doesn't usually have to state what source it comes from or what methods were used to treat it. A 2009 investigation by the U.S. Government Accountability Office found that only "a small percentage" of all bottled water companies give their customers access to the same information about their water that municipal water suppliers are required to provide.

The FDA monitors and inspects water bottling plants, but it considers this job a "low priority" and doesn't do it on any kind of regular schedule. Moreover, if a bottler fails to meet federal safety standards, it can still sell the water. All it has to do is put a statement on the label, such as "contains excessive bacteria" or "excessively radioactive." In 1999, the National Resources Defense Council, an environmental group, tested 1,000 bottles of water from 103 different brands and found that for about one-third of them, at least one sample was over the allowable limits for synthetic organic chemicals, bacteria, or arsenic.

Germs are particularly likely to cause problems in bottled water. As the World Health Organization explains in its 2008 Guidelines for Drinking-Water Quality, "Some microorganisms that are normally of little or no public health significance may grow to higher levels in bottled water." Food Safety News reports that in June 2015, 14 different brands of bottled water had to be recalled because of possible contamination with E. coli bacteria.

Fortunately, no one was sickened by this water, but problems with bottled water aren't always caught in time. The Centers for Disease Control and Prevention lists 14 outbreaks of acute gastrointestinal illness caused by bottled water between 1973 and 2010.

Sustainability

When it comes to taste and safety, bottled water isn't necessarily worse than tap water – it just isn't better. However, when it comes to its environmental impact, tap water is definitely far greener.

The environmental costs of bottled water include the following:

- **Water Scarcity.** Fiji Water isn't the only brand that comes from a place where water resources are limited. Many American brands get their water from drought-ridden California. Arrowhead and Crystal Geyser tap natural springs in the California Mountains, while Aquafina and Dasani draw on the municipal water supply in California cities, according to an investigation by The Desert Sun. In fact, The Desert Sun reports that Nestle Waters North America gets its Arrowhead water from a spring in the San Bernadino National Forest using a permit that officially expired in 1988. To add insult to injury, the companies use still more water in the manufacturing process. A representative of the Coca-Cola Company admitted to Mother Jones that its plants use 1.63 liters of water for every liter of bottled beverages they produce in California – including Dasani bottled water.

* **Toxic Chemicals.** Most water bottles are made from a kind of plastic called polyethylene terephthalate, or PET. Manufacturing this type of plastic produces a variety of toxic chemicals into the air, including nickel, ethyl benzene, ethylene oxide, and benzene. According to a report by the Berkeley Plastics Task Force, making a 16-ounce bottle out of PET creates more than 100 times as much air and water pollution as making the bottle out of glass. Worse still, some of the toxic chemicals in the plastic can leach out over time into the water inside – particularly if the bottle is rinsed and reused.

* **Energy Use.** Bottled water uses energy at every stage of production: treating the water, manufacturing the bottles, filling them, shipping them, and keeping the water cold. The Pacific Institute calculated in 2007 that just producing the bottles for the bottled water Americans drink used the equivalent of more than 17 million barrels of oil. A 2009 Pacific Institute report, published in the peer-reviewed journal Environmental Research Letters, concludes that across its entire life cycle, bottled water takes anywhere from 1,100 to 2,000 times as much energy to produce as tap water.

- **Greenhouse Gas Emissions**. Anything that uses fossil fuels also creates greenhouse gases. The Pacific Institute estimates that the manufacturing of plastic water bottles alone produced more than 2.5 million tons of carbon dioxide in 2006 – not even counting the emissions from shipping the bottles. According to the EPA's Greenhouse Gas Equivalencies Calculator, that gives water bottles a carbon footprint equal to more than half a million passenger vehicles.

- **Packaging Waste**. The Pacific Institute calculates that about 3.8 million tons of PET are used each year to make water bottles – and only about 31% of that PET gets recycled, according to a 2012 EPA fact sheet. The rest ends up in landfills or gets burned (releasing toxic chemicals such as dioxin in the process), or simply gets tossed aside as litter. Many discarded plastic bottles eventually make their way into the oceans, where they can prove deadly to fish, seabirds, and other creatures that swallow them.

Fitting Tap Water Into Your Lifestyle

Despite the many drawbacks of bottled water, a great number of people still feel like they have no real choice about using it. People who live in areas where the local tap water is unsafe or bad-tasting often see bottled water as the only alternative. Other people have no problem drinking tap water at home, but they find it more convenient to carry bottled water when they're out and about, since they can't count on having a tap to get water from everywhere they go.

Fortunately, there are ways to get around these problems. With two simple, inexpensive tools – a water filter and a reusable bottle – you can enjoy tap water that's just as clean, tasty, and convenient to use as bottled water, and far less pricey.

Filter Your Water

If you don't trust your local tap water, or you just don't like the way it tastes, you can filter it to remove impurities. That's exactly what water-bottling companies do when they bottle municipal water, but doing it yourself is a lot cheaper. The Environmental Working Group (EWG), which tested both bottled and tap water in 2008, calculates that using a simple carbon filter – either in a pitcher or attached to your tap – can give you clean, fresh-tasting water for only $0.31 per gallon. That's about one-quarter of the average cost per gallon for bottled water, and less than 5% of what it costs to buy in single-serve bottles.

If you're not sure such a basic filter can deal with your local water, you can find out by consulting the EWG's National Drinking Water Database. Just enter your ZIP Code and the name of your water company to find out what contaminants have been detected in your area's drinking water. Once you know what you need to filter out, you can click on "Get a Water Filter" to find filters that are capable of removing those impurities. Popular options range from a basic Brita water filter pitcher to the Berkey water filtration system.

How is bottled water regulated?

Bottled water was not always standardized. That is, water bottling companies had the liberty to label their bottled water any way they pleased. This all changed in 1996 when the FDA set standards that all bottled water companies were required to follow. Some of the standards included:

- Bottled water from municipal supplies must be clearly labeled as such, unless it is processed sufficiently to be labeled as "distilled" or "purified" water.

- Bottled water must be processed, packaged, shipped, and stored in a safe and sanitary manner and be truthfully and accurately labeled.
- Bottled water must also meet specific FDA quality standards for contaminants.

Is bottled water really healthier than tap water?

One contributing factor to the popularity of bottled water is that people commonly believe that bottled water is "healthier" than tap water is. Calcium (Ca) and magnesium (Mg), in particular, are important minerals we would want in our water. Death rates tend to be lower in areas with tap water containing higher levels of Ca and Mg. It has been shown that deficiencies in magnesium are capable of producing heart disturbances, including 215,000 fatal heart attacks in the U.S. each year, and as many as 20,000,000 fatal heart attacks worldwide!

However, sources say that few brands of bottled water offer a significant amount of minerals. Below is a comparison of calcium and magnesium in bottled and tap water in a few major cities. The numbers represented in this table are the percentages of FDA recommended daily intake per liter for adults.

Bottled Water	%Ca	%Mg	Tap Water	%Ca	%Mg
Crystal Geyser	1	1	San Diego	9	6
Evian	8	6	L.A.	4	4
La Croix	6	6	Houston	4	1
Perrier	9	1	Chicago	4	3
San Pellegrino	20	14	New York	1	0.4
Volvic	1	2	Detroit	3	2

Sources: FDA; city water department; bottled water companies

From these figures, it can be concluded that bottled and tap water can be equally "healthy" in terms of calcium and magnesium content, depending on where you live.

What is the difference between the different types of bottled water anyway?

Mineral water, still water, sparkling water, seltzer water and club soda, sterilized water, and distilled or de-mineralized water. What do all of these have in common? They are all different types of bottled water. So what is the difference?

Mineral water is drawn from an underground source and contains at least 250 ppm of dissolved salts. Whichever minerals are present are what make mineral water what it is. Some minerals that may appear in mineral water include calcium, iron, and sodium.

Still water is water without the "fizz" caused by gas bubbles. Ordinary tap water and bottled water in larger containers are examples of still water.

Sparkling water is water which is carbonated (contains CO_2, producing the "fizz"). It can either be naturally carbonated or mechanically carbonated in a process where CO_2 is added to normal tap water.

Seltzer water is tap water that has been filtered and carbonated. Club soda is seltzer water with added mineral salts.

Sterilized water is used to make baby formula and is also drunk by people with immune-compromised systems. It must be processed to meet FDA's requirements for commercial sterility.

Distilled or de-mineralized water is usually tap water that has been treated to remove nearly all minerals and sodium that occur naturally in water. Natural water usually contains a number of microscopic contaminants, along with dissolved minerals such as calcium and iron. One way to remove these elements from water is to boil it until it changes to steam, a process known as distillation. When this steam is allowed to cool down and condense into liquid form again, the result is a purified form called distilled water. Distilled water should ideally be nothing but hydrogen and oxygen molecules, with a PH level of 7 and no additional gases, minerals or contaminants.

Bottle Maintenance

"What is bottle maintenance?" you ask. After all that you know about tap and bottled water now, if you still think you prefer bottled water, it is important for you to take good care of the bottle from which you drink. Bacteria grow best in warm and moist environments. That means the environment created by an unrefrigerated bottle of water, once the seal has been broken, is the perfect place for bacteria to grow. This produces a plethora of unwanted health risks.

Here are some tips for bottle maintenance. Don't forget to share them with your friends!

- Wipe the seal with a clean cloth after each use.
- Avoid any type of buildup in the bottle cap.
- If your bottle is refillable, make sure it is well cleaned and rinsed before refilling. If possible, recycle the old bottle and obtain a fresh, sterile, sealed bottle.

Sources & References:

Read more : http://www.ehow.com/list_7543970_raw-requirements-plastic-manufacturing-company.html

Read more : http://www.ehow.com/about_5747796_raw-materials-plastic-bottles_.html?ref=Track2&utm_source=ask

United Nations: http://www.unwater.org/water-cooperation2013/water-cooperation/factsandfigures/en/
NPR: http://www.npr.org/2010/12/01/131733493/a-bottledwaterdrama-in-fiji

SDWA:
http://water.epa.gov/lawsreg/rulesregs/sdwa/index.cfm
IBWA: http://www.bottledwater.org/bottled-water-sales-and-consumption-projected-incvrease-2014-expected-be-number-one-packaged-drink

ABC News:
http://www.abcnews.go.com/2020/health/story?id=728070&pages=1

IBWA: http://www.bottledwater.org/economics/red-cost-of-bottled-water

EPA:
http://www.water.epa.gov/drink/guide/upload/book/waterontap_full.pdf

Beverage Marketing Corporation:
http://www.beveragemarketing.com/news-detail.asp?id=260

GMA:
http://www.abcnews.go.com/gma/story?id=126984&page=1
Boston University: http://www.bu.edu/today/2011/bottled-vs-tap-which-tastes-better/

Center for Nutrition Diet and Health:
http://www.udc.edu/docs/causes/online/waterprojecthandout.pdf

Mother Jones: http://www.motherjones.com/blue-marble/2009/07/bottled-waters-can-you-taste-difference

BBC News: http://www.bbc.com/news/uk-33783942
Bottlemania: How Water Went on Sale and Why We Bought It:
http://www.amazon.com

NPR:
http://www.npr.org/templates/story/story.php?storyid=92222327

Safe Drinking Water Act:
http://www.water/epa/gov/lawsregs/rulesregs/sdwa/index.cfm

FDA:
http://www.fda.gov/food/foodborneillnesscontaminants/buystoreservesafefood/ucm077079.htm

Government Accountability Office:
http://www.gao.gov/highlights/d09610high.pdf

National Resources Defense Council:
http://www.nrdc.org/water/drinking/nbw.asp

2008 Guidelines For Drinking-Water Quality:
http://www.who.int/water_sanitation_health/dwq/fulltext.pdf

Centers For Disease Control and Prevention:
http://www.cdc.gov/healthywater/drinking/bottled/

Arrowhead: http://www.nestle-watersna.com/asset-library/documents/ar_eng.pdf

Crystal Geyser: http://www.crystalgeyserasw.com/faqs.html

The Desert Sun:
http://www.desertsun.com/story/news/2015/03/05/bottling-water-california-drought/42389417

Mother Jones:
http://www.motherjones.com/environment/2014/08/bottled-water-california-drought

Berkeley Plastics Task Force: http://ec.electricembers.net/wp-content/uploads/2013/04/ptf_1996.pdf

Toxic chemicals in the plastics:
http://www.moneycrashers.com/dangers-plastic-food-containers-bottles-bisphenol-a/

Pacific Institute: http://pacinst.org/publication/bottled-water-and-energy-a-fact-sheet

Pacific Institute: http://iopscience.iop.org/article/10.1088/1748-9326/4/1/014009/pdf

EPA's Greenhouse Gas Equivalencies Calculator:
http://www2.epa.gov/energy/greenhouse-gas-equivalences-calculator

Carbon Footprint: http://www.moneycrashers.com/carbon-footprint-definition-calculate-reduce/

2012 EPA Fact Sheet:
http://www3.epa.gov/epawaste/nonhaz/municipal/pubs/2012/_msw_fs.pdf

EWG: http://www.ewg.org/research/bottled-water-quality-investigation

National Drinking Water Database: http://www.ewg.org/tap-water/whats-in-your-water.php

Brita Water Filter Pitcher: http://www.amazon.com

Berkey Water Filtration System: http://www.amzaon.com

Chapter 5
Can We Trust Our Municipalities?

I personally feel that it's imperative that we all take our health and wellbeing into our own hands. While it is true that our municipalities adhere to the strict guidelines set forth by the Federal Government, those guidelines have us consuming elements such as chlorine, fluoride, as well as nitrates.

Below is a partial list of contaminates that are included in the water supplies of most US Municipalities. All the containments are considered to be within acceptable Maximum Containment Levels (MCL's).

Containment	Potential Health Effects from Long-Term Exposure above the Maximum Containment Level
Chloramines (As CL2)	Eye/nose irritation, stomach discomfort, anemia
Chlorine (As CL2)	Eye/nose irritation, stomach discomfort
Chlorine dioxide (As CL2)	Anemia in infants and young children, nervous system effects.
Fluoride	Bone disease (pain and tenderness of the bones): Children may get mottled teeth.
Nitrate (measured as Nitrogen)	Infants below the age of six months who drink water-containing nitrate in excess of the Maximum Containment Levels could become seriously ill and, if untreated, may die. Symptoms include shortness of breath and blue-baby syndrome.

How do you learn more about your drinking water?

EPA strongly encourages people to learn more about their drinking water, and to support local efforts to protect the supply of safe drinking water and upgrade the community water system. Your water bill or telephone book's government listings are a good starting point for local information.

Contact your water utility. EPA requires all community water systems to prepare and deliver an annual consumer confidence report (CCR) (sometimes called a water quality report) for their customers by July 1 of each year. If your water provider is not a community water system, or if you have a private water supply, request a copy from a nearby community water system.

Chapter 6
What About Chlorine in our Water Supplies?

What Is Chlorine?

Chlorine is bleach. Adding bleach into our municipal water supplies kills harmful bacteria, and strips our fruits and vegetables of important nutrients.

Drinking Water Treatment:
Why Chlorine is so Very Dangerous

DANGER! Natural organic substances such as fruits, vegetables, and soy products can form dangerous cancer-causing compounds when combined with chlorinated water.

JUST SAY "NO! NO! NO!" TO CHLORINE!!!

Some of nature's most valuable and essential anti-cancer and anti-disease phytochemical nutrients, which are commonly found in food, have been discovered to form deadly cancer-causing substances when consumed or combined with chlorinated tap water. This discovery includes familiar foods including soy, fruits, vegetables, tea, many health products, and some prescriptions.

Recently, a joint study was undertaken in Japan by research scientists at the National Institute of Health Sciences and Shizuoka Prefectural University. They determined that natural organic substances react when exposed to chlorinated tap water, forming dangerous cancer-causing compounds named MX, which stands for "Unknown Mutagen." They are similar to the already well-known and more easily detected cancer causing THMs (trihalomethanes).

Earlier studies by scientists in Finland in 1997 determined that MX is 170 times more deadly than other known toxic by-products of chlorination, and was shown in laboratory studies to damage the thyroid gland as well as cause cancerous tumors.

There is nothing wrong with the organic substances themselves. It is chlorine that is at fault for turning them into the deadly THM and MX cancer cocktail. The reality is that the organic substances have been shown to be highly beneficial combined with alkaline water.

It is certain that the fresh plant foods we eat similarly react with the chlorinated tap water we drink with our meals, creating toxins. This means that fresh fruits and vegetables, green salads, green tea, black tea, herb teas, soy products, vitamins and various health supplements, and even some pharmaceutical drugs all can be implicated in combination with chlorinated water.

The dangerous cancer-causing agents that are produced are extremely toxic in infinitesimal amounts so small and obscure that they are very difficult to detect. Very little chlorine is required.

Many years ago laws were passed making chlorination of water mandatory. Now, the chlorine industry and government agencies must continue their existing policies, because if sudden or drastic changes are made the legal liabilities would be staggering. This predicament could make the tobacco industry scandal seem insignificant in comparison. Educating people about the dangers of chlorine would be admitting to knowledge of the problem, which could invalidate past studies and certainly raise serious legal problems.

Although chlorine has essentially eliminated the risks of waterborne diseases such as typhoid fever, cholera and dysentery, there are many pathogens that are not controlled by chlorine. Better methods of water treatment exist, such as ionization, and many alternatives are already used throughout the world.

This message is of utmost importance to the general public, because chlorine will one day, in the near future, be exposed as a major cause and contributor to cancer and degenerative disease. Chlorine will also be found to be responsible for damaging the body's immune and hormonal systems by mutating the food-based plant estrogens and phytochemicals that support those systems. A healthy immune system should be your first and best line of defense against disease.

What can you do?

Eliminate or reduce all chlorine wherever possible. Don't drink chlorinated tap water. The best way to remove it is to get a reverse osmosis filter, because reverse osmosis also removes fluoride, which is rated a 4/5 on the world poison scales (5 is the highest point). The problem with Reverse Osmosis is that it removes all nutrients from your water. You would then need to add back in the nutrients that our bodies so desperately need. A high quality ionization water machine will provide you with the nutrients needed and rid your water of the chlorine.

Don't bathe in chlorinated water if possible. Filters are available for faucets and shower heads.

The bottom line is that the real culprit is chlorine, not the substances with which it reacts. Many people have larger filter systems installed right on the water line entering their house. Chlorine is everywhere...the ice tea you order at a restaurant was probably made with chlorinated water, your salad leaves may have been washed with chlorinated water...it goes on and on. Many people who read about the dangers of chlorine for the first time are horrified and shocked that this toxic substance is flowing right out of their faucets. But, it is, and knowing about it can only help you to evaluate how you can effectively deal with this toxic addition to daily life.

WATER TEST KITS

If you're wondering whether a water source has chlorine in it, you can purchase water testing kits at your local pool supply store. They're inexpensive and will tell you if that bottled water you're buying is really free of chlorine or not.

I have 3 suggestions:

1. Reduce toxins as much as possible from your daily routine.

2. Supply your body with products that will de-tox and flush existing toxins from your system.

3. Install a good quality ionization water system.

Sources & References:
Toxins: http://www.relfe.com/anti.aging.html

Chapter 7
What About Fluoride in Our Water?

What is Fluoride; Is it good or bad for us?

Fluoride is a very toxic poison that is not good to be ingested, especially in large quantities. There is historical evidence of the damage that has been done on the people that have consumed it. New evidence has shown that the addition of fluoride in our water supplies is actually having adverse effects on consumers, especially on young children.

Why did our government believe that fluoride would be helpful?

According to the Environmental Protection Agency, fluoride is voluntarily added to some drinking water systems as a public health measure for reducing the incidence of cavities among the treated population. The decision to fluoridate a water supply is made by the state or local municipality, and is not mandated by EPA or any other Federal entity. The Centers for Disease Control and Prevention (CDC) provides recommendations about the optimal levels of fluoride in drinking water in order to prevent tooth decay.

ADA study confirms dangers of fluoridated water, especially for babies

(NaturalNews) Advocates of fluoridated water insist that the chemical additive is good for teeth, but actual science routinely shows otherwise, including a new study published in the *Journal of the American Dental Association* confirming fluoride as a toxic substance that actually destroys teeth, particularly those of developing young children and babies.

When people are exposed to excessive levels of fluoride through sources like drinking water, foods and beverages and even swallowed toothpaste, it often results in a condition known as dental fluorosis. The internal uptake of fluoride into teeth over time causes their enamel to become mottled and discolored, the end result being damaged teeth that have essentially rotted from the inside out. I dated a man that had this unfortunate condition. It didn't end well.

Dr. Steven Levy, D.D.S., and his team found during their study that "fluoride intakes during each of the first four years (of a child's life) were individually significantly related to fluorosis on maxillary central incisors, with the first year more important." They went on to warn that "infant formulas reconstituted with higher fluoride water can provide 100 to 200 times more fluoride than breast milk, or cow's milk."

In other words, young children have the highest risk of severe tooth damage from fluoride, especially those that are six months of age or younger, a time during which children's blood-brain barriers have not fully formed. Even low ingestion levels cause the direct depositing of fluoride into the teeth, brain and other bodily tissues and organs which, besides causing fluorosis, also causes disorders of the brain and nervous system, kidneys and bones.

And the American Dental Association (ADA) has known that fluoride exposure causes dental fluorosis since at least 2006, but the group has done nothing to warn the 200 million Americans that live in communities with fluoridated water to avoid its use in babies and infants. Many dentists still recommend that children and adults not only drink fluoridated water, but even advise parents to add fluoride drops to their children's drinking water if the family lives in un-fluoridated areas or drinks private well water.

Fluoride causes serious health problems

In 2006, a study published in *The Lancet* identified fluoride as "an emerging neurotoxic substance" that causes severe brain damage. The National Research Council (NRC) wrote that "it is apparent that fluorides have the ability to interfere with the functions of the brain and the body by direct and indirect means."

About a month later, another study published in *Environmental Health Perspectives* found a definitive link between fluoride intake and reduced IQ levels, indicating once again that fluoride intake causes cognitive damage.

At Harvard University, researchers identified a link between fluoride and bone cancer. Published 14 years after it began, the study found that the highest rates of osteosarcoma, a fatal form of bone cancer, were occurring most in populations drinking fluoridated water. The findings confirmed those of a prior government study back in 1990 that involved fluoride-treated rats.

Kidney disease is another hallmark of fluoride poisoning. Multiple animal studies have found that fluoride levels as low as 1 part per million (ppm) -- which is the amount added to most fluoridated water systems -- cause kidney damage. And a Chinese study found that children exposed to slightly higher fluoride levels had biological markers in their blood, indicative of kidney damage.

The NRC has also found that fluoride impairs proper thyroid function and debilitates the endocrine system. Up until the 1970s, fluoride was used in Europe as a thyroid-suppressing medication because it lowers thyroid function. Many experts believe that widespread hypothyroidism today is a result of overexposure to fluoride.

Since fluoride is present in most municipal water supplies in North America, it is absurd to even suggest that parents avoid giving it to their young children. How are parents supposed to avoid it unless they install a whole-house ionization water filtration system? And even if families install such a system, fluoride is found in all sorts of food and beverages, not to mention that it is absorbed through the skin every time people wash their hands with or take a shower in fluoridated water. Perhaps these are some of the reasons why the ADA has said nothing about the issue, despite the findings.

There simply is no legitimate reason to fluoridate water. Doing so forcibly medicates an entire population with a carcinogenic, chemical drug. There really is no effective way to avoid it entirely, and nobody really knows how much is ingested or absorbed on a daily basis because exposure is too widespread to calculate. But political pressure and bad science have continued to justify water fluoridation in most major cities, despite growing mountains of evidence showing its dangers.

Ending water fluoridation is a difficult task, but concerted efforts by citizens, local authorities, and even dentists, have resulted in some significant victories. To learn more about fluoride, check out the Fluoride Action Network (FAN):

http://www.fluoridealert.org

Sources & References:

Ethan A. Huff, staff writer for Natural News

Learn more:
http://www.naturalnews.com/030123_fluoride_babies.html#ix
zz3qMTqrmYp

http://www.naturalnews.com/study/html

http://naturalnews.com/floridated_water/html

http://www.prnewswire.com/news-releases/pare...

http://jada.ada.org/cgi/content/abstract/141

http://www.fluoridealert.org/health/cancer/

Chapter 8
What are Environmental Protection Agency (EPA) drinking water regulations for nitrates?

What are nitrates?

Nitrates and nitrites are nitrogen-oxygen chemical units, which combine with various organic and inorganic compounds.

Uses for nitrate

The greatest use of nitrates is as a fertilizer. Once taken into the body, nitrates are converted to nitrites.

What are nitrate's health effects?

Infants below six months who drink water containing nitrate in excess of the maximum contaminant level (MCL) could become seriously ill and, if untreated, may die. Symptoms include shortness of breath and blue baby syndrome.

This health effects language is not intended to catalog all possible health effects for nitrate. Rather, it is intended to inform consumers of some of the possible health effects associated with nitrate in drinking water when the rule was finalized.

In 1974, Congress passed the Safe Drinking Water Act. This law requires EPA to determine the level of contaminants in drinking water at which no adverse health effects are likely to occur. These non-enforceable health goals, based solely on possible health risks and exposure over a lifetime with an adequate margin of safety, are called maximum contaminant level goals (MCLG). Contaminants are any physical, chemical, biological or radiological substances or matter in water.

The MCLG for nitrate is 10 mg/L or 10 ppm. EPA has set this level of protection based on the best available science to prevent potential health problems. EPA has set an enforceable regulation for nitrate, called a maximum contaminant level (MCL), at 10 mg/L or 10 ppm. MCLs are set as close to the health goals as possible, considering cost, benefits and the ability of public water systems to detect and remove contaminants using suitable treatment technologies. In this case, the MCL equals the MCLG, because analytical methods or treatment technology do not pose any limitation.

The Phase II Rule, the regulation for nitrate, became effective in 1992. The Safe Drinking Water Act requires EPA to periodically review the national primary drinking water regulation for each contaminant and revise the regulation, if appropriate. EPA reviewed nitrate as part of the Six Year Review and determined that the 10 mg/L or 10-ppm MCLG and 10 mg/L or 10 ppm MCL for nitrate are still protective of human health.

States may set more stringent drinking water MCLGs and MCLs for nitrates than EPA.

How does nitrate get into my drinking water?

The major sources of nitrates in drinking water are runoff from fertilizer use; leaking from septic tanks, sewage; and erosion of natural deposits.

A federal law called the Emergency Planning and Community Right to Know Act (EPCRA) requires facilities in certain industries, which manufacture, process, or use significant amounts of toxic chemicals, to report annually on their releases of these chemicals. For more information on the uses and releases of chemicals in your state, contact the Community Right-to-Know Hotline: (800) 424-9346.

How will I know if nitrate is in my drinking water?

When routine monitoring indicates that nitrate levels are above the MCL, your water supplier must take steps to reduce the amount of nitrate so that it is below that level. Water suppliers must notify their customers as soon as practical, but no later than 24 hours after the system learns of the violation. Additional actions, such as providing alternative drinking water supplies, may be required to prevent serious risks to public health.

If your water comes from a household well, check with your health department or local water systems that use ground water for information on contaminants of concern in your area.

How will nitrate be removed from my drinking water?

The following treatment method(s) have proven to be effective for removing nitrate to below 10 mg/L or 10 ppm: ion exchange (ionization water machine), reverse osmosis, electro dialysis.

How do I learn more about my drinking water?

EPA strongly encourages people to learn more about their drinking water, and to support local efforts to protect the supply of safe drinking water and upgrade the community water system. Your water bill or telephone book's government listings are a good starting point for local information.

Contact your water utility. EPA requires all community water systems to prepare and deliver an annual consumer confidence report (CCR) (sometimes called a water quality report) for their customers by July 1 of each year. If your water provider is not a community water system, or if you have a private water supply, request a copy from a nearby community water system.

Chapter 9
Finding The Right Water Ionizer

The purpose of this chapter is to help you make an informed decision about which ionizer to purchase.

There are three very important things to consider:

1. You should consider your health goals.
2. You should consider your budget and lifestyle.
3. You should choose a quality unit from a reliable manufacturer.

If health is your primary goal, are you trying to improve your health, increase athletic performance or to slow down the aging process? Whatever the case, you will want a high-performance water ionizer. High-performance water ionizers can supply high levels of alkaline water (9.5+ pH). This level of alkalinity has a high level of anti-oxidant potential or ORP (oxygen reduction potential) and high levels of alkaline mineral hydrates. Both properties are very important for achieving your health and or athletic performance goals.

If budget and lifestyle are of more importance, then focus on ionizers within your price range or budget. But don't skimp on quality. You may need to eliminate some of the bells and whistles of some units and just stick with the basics of good alkaline water.

You should also consider the placement of the ionizer. The options available are either a counter top or under the sink.

Do you travel? If so look, for ionizer companies that offer various size bottles as well as travel pitchers. Once you become accustomed to drinking alkaline/ionized water you won't want to be without it for even one day.

As you've learned from previous chapters, alkaline water should not be stored or used with regular plastic bottles. The detoxification properties of alkaline water can leech the chemical properties of the plastic into the water.

Choose a quality unit. The investment in your health should last a lifetime. Some important issues to consider are warranties, return policies, trial periods and after care.

The main elements in an ionizer are:

1. The customized filters designed to remove contaminants are the most overlooked and under-considered components of any water ionizer. Most people don't understand that when water is passing through an ionizer an efficient power system with high quality plates is essential. The first medium that it comes into contact with is the filter(s). If an ionizer has poor filtration, you will essentially be drinking dirty and potentially harmful ionized water.

Here are a few tips for you to follow:

- If a water ionizer has only one filter, cross if off your list. There are too many dual filter water ionizers on the market today to even consider a single filter unit.

- Look for large filters. The physical size of the filter matters just as much as what is inside it. Since the water travels through the filter from top to bottom, I found that the longer the filter, the better the filtration.

- Insist on ceramic. Ceramic filters are a serious game-changer for the water ionization industry. Only made available in the last 5 years, ceramic filters are super-effective against bacteria, protozoa, and microbial cysts. You don't want to drink those bad boys.

- Consider filter price. While buying one of those units with the inexpensive filters may seem appealing, inexpensive filters mean inexpensive filter content, and less of it. Top brands are charging up to $30-$40 more for a set of replacement filters. There are justified reasons for higher filter prices, and in this particular case - you really do get what you pay for. Getting the best filters possible shouldn't be much of a decision at all.

- Use pre filters when necessary. All of the top-rated companies have many pre-filter options that can help solve almost all source water challenges. From hard water to soft water and everything in between, a reputable ionizer company will have a solution for you. Be sure to discuss any concerns that you have regarding your water type and ask the ionizer company of your choice to run a water report so you can get the pre-filters that you need.

2. The plates must be titanium, coated with platinum. You should insist on a platinum coating with a thickness of at least 20 microns. The style of the plate will directly affect the performance of the machine. The number of plates in a water ionizer is critically important. Perhaps the only thing more important than the number of plates is the size, type and quality of the plates. The main function of the plates inside of a water ionizer is to restructure the water and separate it into acidic and alkaline streams. This restructuring and separation requires high amounts of electricity. The goal is to conduct as much electricity as

possible and to utilize as much of the plate surface area as possible in order to gain the most effect on the water. The plates can be found inside the water cell, which is the heart of any water ionizer. Plates are made of various types of metals, with the highest quality plates made of titanium and then coated several times with platinum. The amount of platinum used on the plates can greatly affect the price of a water ionizer since the going rate for platinum is ever-increasing.

3. Efficient power is very important. Water ionizers make alkaline water by using electro magnetism to separate the alkaline minerals from the acidic substances in the water. The more power a ionizer has the stronger the alkaline water it can make. In general, you want an ionizer that has 400 watts or more of power.

4. Where will the ionizer be placed? Some ionizers are designed to work on the counter top, others are designed to work under the sink. The best ionizers are convertible water ionizers. Convertible ionizers are a better choice because they give you the flexibility to choose.

5. My ionizer is on my counter top. It makes for easy access when I want to switch between acid or alkaline water. Plus, it matches my appliances nicely.

6. High quality water ionizers come with long warranties of 5 plus years. Get to know the company that you're planning to do business with. When you buy a water ionizer you're establishing a long-term relationship. You will need to contact them for replacement filters and for warranty service. Find out how long they've been in business; 10+ years is best.

How Does a Water Ionizer Work?

There are three main elements in a water ionizer that combine together to create delicious high pH and anti-oxidant rich water. First, the unit must eliminate water contaminants while preserving the minerals. Second, the power system delivers a range of watts depending on which model and manufacturer. Third, is high quality plates made with high quality materials? The combination of plates and power equals the efficiency at which the system separates the ions in the water. The greater the efficiency at separating the ions, the stronger the alkaline water will be in pH and ORP (oxygen reduction potential). This process is known as electro dialysis.

Here is what Ray Kurzweil, author, inventor and futurist, has to say about the benefits of alkaline water. "There are more benefits to "alkaline water" than simply the alkalinity or pH. The most important feature of alkaline water produced by a water ionizer is its oxidation reduction potential (ORP). Water with a high negative ORP is of particular value in its ability to neutralize oxygen free radicals."

What is and What is Not Filtered Out?

Water ionizer's internal filters are designed primarily to filter chlorine and sediments out of your water. Most water ionizers use activated carbon filters, which reduce chlorine and some metals in your water supply.

Activated carbon filters don't remove all contaminants. The contaminates that are not removed by activated carbon filters are:

- Fluoride
- Some heavy metals including arsenic
- Prescription drug residues
- Nitrates
- Chemicals from fracking, and many others.

If you determine, after a water analysis that these elements need be addressed, consider even further filtration methods to address those concerns. I had to install an additional unit to address the high amount of iron in our well water. Our water is crystal clear now and it tastes pure.

Chapter 10
The Top Six Water Ionizers

The Four Most Important Factors When Buying a Water Ionizer

Plates the most important element
Plate Details, Coating, Material, Quality and Thickness

The ionizer plates are the most expensive part of a water ionizer because they are coated with platinum- a precious metal that costs over $1,600 per ounce. The platinum coating on the plates should be 20 microns thick, anything less isn't enough to be reliable. High quality ionizers will have eight coats of platinum on their plates. It's expensive to put eight coats of platinum on the plates, - but that's why high quality ionizers come with lifetime warranties.

Types of Plates

Flat plates

Used in the first ionizers from the 1950's to current water ionizers, these plates are just how the name describes them - Flat.

These are being touted as most reliable by some proponents.

Mesh plates

These plates are a more recent development compared to the flat plates. Research and development found that creating more edges on the water ionizer plates created a stronger water during ionization due to the Faraday Effect: Electricity likes to travel along edges, rather than on flat surfaces. Tests find that these plates deliver 10-15% better performance in pH and ORP.

Hybrid plates

These plates are simply flat plates with large holes cut into them.

Our reviewers report that water flow is increased compared to other plates.

Grid plates

The newest innovation in water ionizer plate technology, these plates combine the strength of flat plates with the performance of the Mesh plates.

These heavy duty plates are often used in commercial water ionizer applications.

How do they compare?

Grid Plates vs. Mesh Plates	Grid Plates vs. Hybrid Plates	Hybrid Plates vs. Flat Plates
GRID plates are heavy duty plates that combine the benefit of MESH plates with the durability of plated designed for commercial and industrial water ionizers. They are three times stronger than MESH plates, and will out-perform flat plates and Hybrid plates.	Grid plates are stronger than Hybrid plates, and they give 10 - 15% higher pH levels and antioxidant ORP levels than hybrid Plates. Hybrid plates don't offer any real improvement. You will find hybrid plates in cheaper ionizers because they save the manufacturer money.	Hybrid plates perform about the same as flat plates. They are used in some cheaper ionizers because they are not as expensive to manufacture as Grid or MESH plates.

How many plates do I need?

The more high-quality, large plates you have, matched with an SMPS high output power system, the more optimized your water will be. This means more alkaline mineral hydrates, better pH performance and higher levels of antioxidant potential.

Also, the number of plates an ionizer has affects the water flow rate of the ionizer. Flow rate increases with the number of plates simply because the more plates you have, the more space you have for water to flow through the ionization chamber.

The Number of Plates Affects Ionizer Quality

Ultimate quality machines	13 plates
Advanced quality machines	11 plates
Top quality ionizers	9 plates
Mid range systems	7 plates
Entry level machines	5 plates
Avoid machines with	3 plates

What size of plates are best?

Many ionizer manufacturers will argue that bigger is better, and this is true up to a point. Large plates are better if there is an adequate power supply to power them. This is why I recommended earlier that you choose an ionizer with at least 550 watts of power. Underpowered water ionizers often need chemical additives that come with potential side effects.

Safety Concerns In Cheap Ionizers

Here are a few of the dangerous ways that cheap water ionizer manufacturers cut corners:

Chinese and Taiwanese companies often cut costs by putting a minimal coating of Platinum on the Titanium plates. Certified lab tests shows that one company, "Air, Water, Life" (Real Spirit) uses no Platinum and this is why the cost is so low. Beware.

Platinum Plates

Imagine buying a car where every part was made by the lowest bidder.

A cheap car will quickly fall apart and might not even be safe to drive.

The same is true with cheap water ionizers. When every part is made as cheap as possible, the manufacturer compromises on the safety of the unit and the safety of your family with inferior parts being used, and the machine's reliability.

The size, type, material and number of plates is what matters the most. Choose a 9-plate or 11-plate unit with solid/mesh hybrid plates that are at least 7"x4" (don't skimp on this). Make sure that the ionizer plates are made from medical grade, strengthened titanium that is dipped multiple times in platinum.

FILTRATION - The unit must have 2 filters and they must be Ultra filters only. No exceptions! Make sure the company offers pre-filters for unique water types like well water and soft water, etc.

HIGHER POWER MEANS SAFE DRINKING WATER - A 9-plate water ionizer with at least 550 watts will produce super pH levels and ORP levels without adding chemicals. An 11-plate ionizer will need 750 watts; no exceptions. Do not buy a unit with a chemical injection port that adds a salt or saline solution unless you are looking to make a form of bleach! Himalayan salts sound exotic, but not when you want pure and healthy ionized water.

WARRANTY AND TRIAL PERIOD - Tyent USA is the only company that offers a zero-stipulation lifetime warranty and a 75-day trial. Why settle for less?

	Tyent	Kangen®	Chanson	Jupiter	Air Water Life	Life Ionizer	Category Winner
Maximum Number of Plates	11	7	7	9	7	13	Tyent, Life Ionizer
Dual Ultra Filtration	YES	NO	NO	YES	NO	YES	Tyent, Jupiter, Life Ionizer
Maximum Wattage	750	230	150	80	200	504	Tyent
Turbo Mode Availability	YES	NO	NO	NO	NO	NO	Tyent
Lifetime Warranty	YES	NO	NO	NO	NO	YES	Tyent, Life ionizer
Highest ORP	Up To -1050	Up To -850	Up To -780	Up To -800	Up To -750	Up To -812	Tyent
Made in Korea or Japan	YES	YES	NO	YES	NO	YES	Tyent, Kangen®, Jupiter, Life Ionizer
Chemical Free	YES	NO	NO	NO	YES	YES	Tyent, Air Water Life, Life Ionizer
Solid Mesh Hybrid Plates	YES	NO	NO	NO	YES	NO	Tyent, Air Water Life
SMPS Plus Power Supply	YES	NO	NO	NO	NO	YES	Tyent, Life Ionizer

As you can see, Tyent is the top choice in every category. Tyent includes every important feature you should be looking for when purchasing a water ionizer. I personally own the Kangen® Ionizer and, when I purchased it, it was the top of the line in Ionizers. But time brings about a change in all areas of life. I recently moved to an area where only well water is available to my family and me. The soil is full of iron, so additional filtration has become an area of concern.

Always consider the area in which you live and the source and contents of the water you have available. Using a Tyent Ionizer with municipal water sources is an excellent combination.

My next purchase of an ionizer will be with a Tyent Ionizer. Consider the attributes that I have mentioned above and decide what is best for you and your circumstances.

You may contact me at Patricia@patriciaawyatt.com for possible discounts on the unit you choose no matter your choice.

TIPS ON HOW TO REALLY SAVE MONEY ON A WATER IONIZER

Top Tip: Keep Your Eyes Open for Great Water Ionizer Sales!

Insist on a A+ Rating from the Better Business Bureau, which will ensure that the company sells only top-rated water ionizers and that they stand behind quality.

Buy medical-grade, platinum-coated titanium plates only. Permelec plates are the best. That way, you can rest assured that you have a lifetime of safe ionized water.

Shop sales! Many manufacturers, including Tyent, offer sales where you could save $1,000 or more! Email me at Patricia@patriciaawyatt.com for discount pricing!

Only buy machines with the following water ionizer certifications.

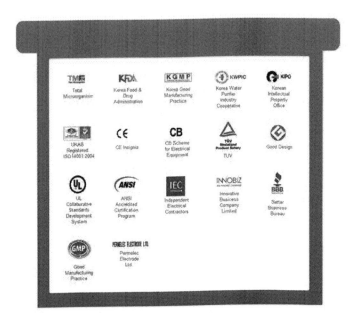

I truly hope that this information has been helpful in helping you to realize the health and nutritional benefits of drinking alkaline water as well as consuming an alkaline diet. The proper pH balance within your body will help to fight off many of diseases and ailments that many suffer from today. I know that my family and I have noticed a tremendous benefit. I take great pride in the fact that at 66 years of age, I'm not on any medicinal prescriptions only a supplement regime agreed upon between me and my Naturopath doctor who, unfortunately is not taking any more patients.

To your continued good health.

Patricia

Chapter 11
Testimonials

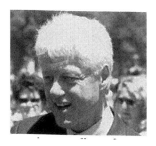

BILL CLINTON
Former President

Mr. Clinton tells us that not only has he lost 24 lbs., but his whole metabolism has changed as a result of this diet.

Mr. Clinton goes on to say that "82% of the people since 1986 who have gone on a plant based, no meat, and no dairy diet have begin to heal themselves. Their arterial blockage breaks up, the calcium deposit around their heart breaks up."

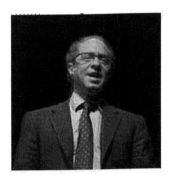

RAY KURZWEIL
Author, Inventor & Futurist

"There are more benefits to "alkaline water" than simply the alkalinity or pH. The most important feature of alkaline water produced by a water Ionizer is its oxidation reduction potential (ORP). Water with a high negative ORP is of particular value in its ability to neutralize oxygen free radicals."

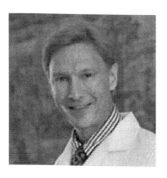

DR. DON COLBERT
N.Y. Times Best Selling Author

"I have had countless numbers of patients with painful osteoarthritis on many different medications for arthritis.

Many have been pain free within a couple of months after adjusting their urine pH to 7.0 to 7.5 by consuming adequate amounts of alkaline water and alkaline foods. As a result, many are able to go off of their medications."

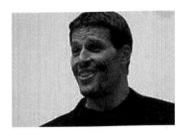

ANTHONY ROBBINS
Inspirational Psychologist

"Alkalize your body and live a healthier, more energized, and ultimately more fulfilling life. Our acid-alkaline balance is a baseline determinant of our physical health. When you break your old eating patterns, you will find yourself getting back to the real you, filled with the vitality and energy that your desire and deserve."

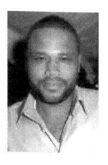

ANTHONY ANDERSON
Professional Actor

"My demanding schedule means sometimes I'm forced to put myself on the back-burner, but the first time I tasted Alkaline water I knew I needed a machine of my own. I found and purchased a Life Ionizer, now it travels absolutely everywhere with me and I drink it every day. I love it!"

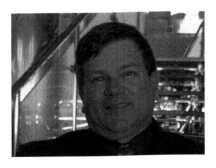

DAVID WYATT
Retired Robotics Engineer

"I once thought that water was, well.... just water. I also thought it was my fate to always be sick. Once I learned about alkaline water and the benefits, there in my life changed. I started drinking high alkaline water (9.5pH) and found that I had more energy, I rarely got sick, and problems I already had went away, such as high blood pressure. I also discovered that high alkaline water taste better. We all benefit from high alkaline water. I highly recommend a high intake of alkaline water to everyone I meet. This is one subject I find it difficult to stay quiet about. Please join me in a healthier life".

Disclaimer: Results may not be typical nor expected for every consumer.

"The body aches and pains have just disappeared in the months I've been drinking this water"

"What I notice most is that the body aches and pains have just disappeared in the months I've been drinking this water. I had been nearly incapacitated with back and leg pain, which had also kept me awake at night. That is now completely gone and I feel better than I have in years.

Also, people around me get sick and I take care of them, but I never seem to come down with it anymore.

I gave some to my daughter who lives in the city and has terrible water. When we added the Adya Clarity, there was quite a bit of gunk left in the bottom of the glass. She no longer buys bottled water now! She also pre-filters before adding the Adya, just so it takes less to clean it up.

I never want to be without this wonderful product. For so many years I craved a simple, clean, pure glass of water to drink instead of the terrible dead, contaminated stuff available, even in bottles. I now have it, and I value this as an absolute treasure."

Thank you,
Linda Hensley

Disclaimer: Results may not be typical nor expected for every consumer.

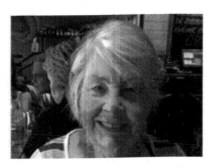

Edith Jones

"I have for a long time found it uneasy to drink water directly from the tap. I have always had to mix it with some juice or other. The water we have here in South Wales, UK looks very good and clear, it does however have a taste of chlorine and God knows what else is being used to clean the water.

I usually put my tap water into a big glass jar with the Adya Clarity and let it stand for at least 12 hours, after that I pour it into a bigger glass vessel. As I pour it into the other glass vessel slowly and carefully, the impurities, becomes clear to see left at the bottom. It is quite a surprise when the water otherwise looks clear and good.

When I do the same without Adya Clarity added, no impurities become visible. Drinking water today is a joy and I feel lucky that I do not have to drink the impurities which I now know are there in the tap water.

A friend of mine came to stay with me for a few days; she immediately noticed the fresh taste of water.

I bought the Adya Clarity because it appealed to me to be able to drink pure fresh water.

Thank you very much for this wonderful discovery. Although my gunk is very fine, I will be sending you a picture of it from my iPad.

The bluish strike in the picture is the gunk. It is very fine. I had to tilt the bowl to make it visible. It can best be seen when the bowl is held in the air, but no one here to give a hand.

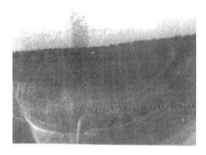

Disclaimer: Results may not be typical nor expected for every consumer.

Dr. A.F.M.

"After a lot of troubles I have send you one photo the first bottle is tap water the second is water from Brita jug filter still dirty, the third is the most pure water Adya Clarity in my jug 2L of it and you can`t see it. The Water is crystal clear and it taste so good. My benefit I am been cleaned from the inside out I see evidence on my skin I feel much stronger thank you regards Alide."

Disclaimer: Results may not be typical nor expected for every consumer.

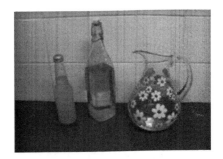

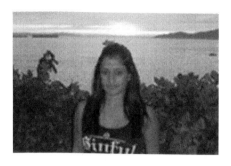

Monisha Jassi

"My name is Monisha Jassi and I have been using Adya Clarity for 3 months now. I add the drops to a jug of tap water at night and in the morning I can see tiny particles of all the yucky stuff that is in the tap water floating around the bottom of the jug. I love the taste of the water, I also clean my fruits and veggies with it. I give it to my plants and my pet. Here is a picture I took of the contaminants at the bottom of my glass after adding Adya Clarity.

Thanks for this great tasting and super easy method of cleaning my water."

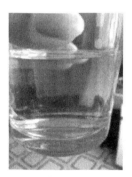 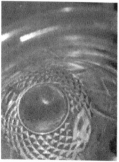

Disclaimer: Results may not be typical nor expected for every consumer.

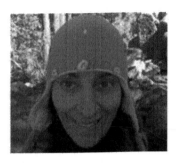

Silvia Berglas

"We've been using Adya Clarity for several years now. Whenever we feel unwell we add Adya Clarity to the water we drink.

Apart from the water tasting so much better, we have noticed that whenever we do that we heal a lot quicker, whether it's a headache, or flu, or a cold. It's even been helpful with food poisoning.
I even use it for my animals, when they have stomach problems, and they love t sip up the water and improve within a very short time. My kids sometimes ask for water with Adya Clarity in it, just because it tastes so much better, and that's even though we have a house water filter that filters the water twice."

Disclaimer: Results may not be typical nor expected for every consumer.

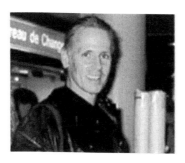

James Justice, Clearwater, FL

"I have been using Adya Clarity for over six months. Before, I drank bottled water exclusively, but often felt bloated and sluggish. Also, I felt like drinking water stored in plastic might be creating more harm to my body than good.

Since switching to Adya Clarity, I feel lighter and brighter. I feel the water I am drinking is helping my body rid itself of stored toxins and contaminants, just like it does with tap water.

When I see the orange residue in the unit, I'm really grateful I found this wonderful water enhancing system."

Disclaimer: Results may not be typical nor expected for every consumer.

Just take a look at this list of Alkaline Water Drinkers:

Jay-Z
Donald Trump
Demi Moore
Steven Tyler (4 machines)
Brad Pitt
Magic Johnson (8 machines)
Jack Nicholson
Chris Daughtry
Bill Gates
Jennifer Lopez
Carlos Santana
Jillian Michaels
Earth, Wind & Fire
Conan O'Brian
Toby Keith
Ron Perlman
Phil Michelson
Roger Daultry
Bodybuilders Big Dan Hill
Yankees

Beyoncé
Bobby P.
Aston Kutcher
Angelina Jolie
Janet Jackson
The Obamas
Steven Seagal
Sammy Hagar
Rohan Marley
Martha Stewart
Elton John
George Lopez
Chuck Norris
Chris Angel
John Mayer
Sly Stallone
Chilean Miners
Cindie Blackman
Wade Lightheart
Lakers

Also endorsed by the American Anti-Cancer Institute and more.

Why are so many celebrities drinking alkaline water? Simple…. They need to maintain their performance, health and beauty! That's why.

Join the growing number of people concerned enough to do something to help ensure a long and quality filled life.

Drink alkaline/ionized mineral water!

About The Author

Patricia Phillips-Wyatt was born in Los Angeles, California. She attended California State University where she obtained a Bachelor of Science degree in Business Administration. She attended National University, La Jolla, California where she earned a Masters Degree in Education Administration. She considers herself a lifetime learner in the areas of Holistic herbal medical solutions, which includes the use of Essential Oils (www.yngliving.com) for healthy remedies.

Patricia Phillips-Wyatt has been passionate about the water we drink since 1991. She became a distributor and installer of NSA Water purification devices and learned some valuable lessons regarding the water quality of the Municipal principalities entrusted with providing quality water for residents. It was during this period that many people, including Patricia herself, really started to notice she didn't like or enjoy the taste of the water coming from our faucets.

In 2003 she learned and saw for herself the difference a water ionizer could make in the pH level of the water. She discovered that one of her favorite bottled water sources was quite acidic which in turn caused oxidation to occur within the body. Oxidation, as she learned was a major cause of the breakdown in the functionality of our cells. This is also why so many Naturopath and Holistic practitioners (and to be fair, many informed medical practitioners), began stressing the importance of consuming anti-oxidants to stay healthy. If it weren't for our consumption of food and drink products that cause oxidation within our bodies, there would be no need to consume foods with high anti-oxidant properties (You'll learn more about the oxidation reduction potential (ORP) within chapter 9.

It was in 2003 that Patricia purchased her first Ionizer water machine. That machine was a Kangen® SD501 by Enagic®. She could tell the difference immediately. The taste was actually a pure clean taste unlike anything that had previously been experienced since she was a kid. Patricia has been an avid advocate of this technology since that time.

Since 2003 many enhancements have taken place in the technology of the machines and believe that as of this writing I have found the best unit on the market. See the chapter on The Top Six Water Ionizers.

As an educator for over 30 years she couldn't in all good conscience keep this valuable and possible life saving information to herself. Teaching is also one of her main passions.

For information call Patricia at 919-888-1981 or email her at Patricia@patriciaawyatt.com.

https://www.facebook.com/AlkalineWaterBook/
https://www.instagram.com/PatTheWaterLady
https://www.linkedin.com/in/patricia-wyatt-64b311125

Made in the USA
Lexington, KY
15 April 2017